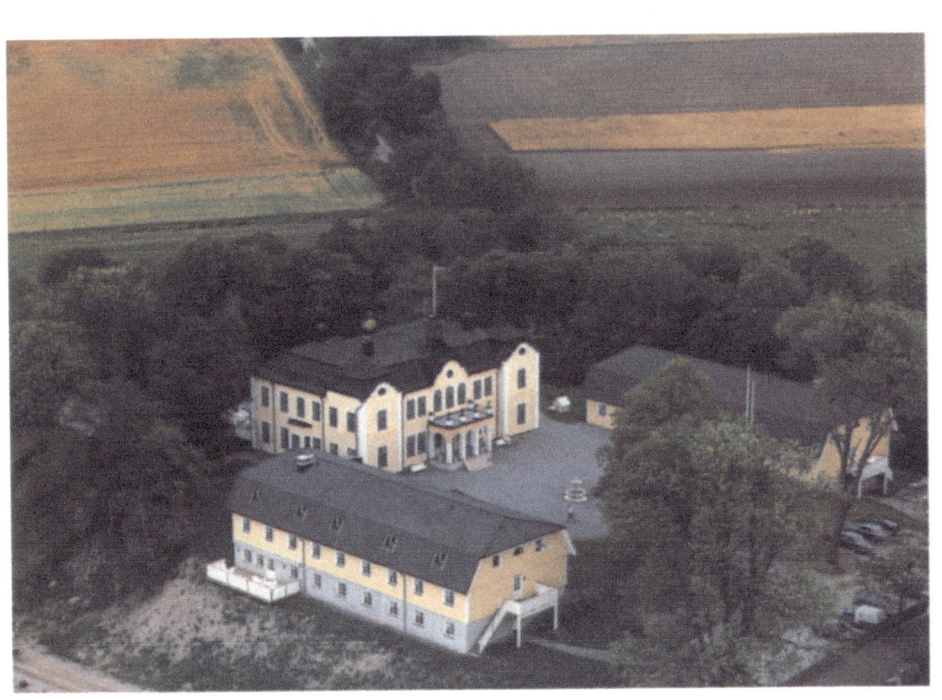

Non-Opioid Analgesics in the Treatment of Acute Pain

Johannesbergs Slott, Sweden, March 14, 1996

Springer Basel AG

A CIP catalogue record for this book is available from the Library of Congress, Washington, D.C., USA

Deutsche Bibliothek – Cataloging-in-Publication Data

Non-opioid analgesics in the treatment of acute pain : Johannesbergs Slott, Sweden, March 14th, 1996 – Basel ; Boston ; Berlin : Birkhäuser, 1997
ISBN 978-3-7643-5680-4   ISBN 978-3-0348-8869-1 (eBook)
DOI 10.1007/978-3-0348-8869-1

1997 Springer Basel AG
Originally published by Birkhäuser Verlag in 1997

Printed on acid-free paper produced from chlorine-free pulp. TCF ∞
ISBN 978-3-7643-5680-4

9 8 7 6 5 4 3 2 1

Contents

Introduction

Dipyrone is widely acknowledged to be an effective antipyretic analgesic with an additional intrinsic spasmolytic activity. It has stood the test of time over the last 75 years in many clinical settings throughout the world. Some 20 years ago, however, concern arose over the implications of isolated reports of agranulocytosis following use of dipyrone. Based on these initial cases the Swedish authorities ordered the withdrawal of the drug from the market. Subsequently, dipyrone has been subjected to extensive comparative epidemiological and clinical studies. The results of these investigations have allayed the earlier concerns and have shown dipyrone to be a versatile analgesic drug with an overall risk of serious adverse events lower than most other non-opioid analgesics. Based on these results, the Swedish authorities (Låkemedelsverket) have approved the reintroduction of dipyrone to clinical use as a valuable contribution to pain treatment. In connection with this further milestone in the story of the drug, a symposium was held in Stockholm on March 14, 1996, under the chairmanship of Professor N. Rawal to review the current understanding of the action, efficacy and safety of dipyrone.

The highlights of this Hoechst symposium emphasize particularly the therapeutic basis for the use of dipyrone in the modern treatment of acute post-operative pain.

Mode of action of dipyrone

Professor K. Brune, M.D.
Erlangen, Germany

Most non-opioid analgesic drugs are inhibitors of cyclo-oxygenase, the enzyme catalysing the formation of prostaglandins (PGs). The local inhibition of inflammatory prostaglandins is considered to be the main mechanism of action of the non-steroidal anti-inflammatory drugs (NSAIDs). The PGs are able to activate so-called "sleeping" or normally unresponsive nociceptors, which sense painful stimuli at sites of inflammation and it is the suppression of this peripheral nociceptor sensitization which contributes to the analgesic action of the NSAIDs.

Dipyrone and its active metabolites are weak inhibitors of cyclo-oxygenase and therefore do not exhibit peripheral anti-inflammatory activity. This was shown in humans in our institute using experimentally-induced pain. Both NSAIDs and dipyrone blocked the pain, but only NSAIDs prevented the inflammatory increase in local blood flow.

Unlike NSAIDs, dipyrone, the active metabolite of which is non-acidic, *does* enter the central nervous system where it has been shown to inhibit hypothalamic PG synthesis leading to antipyresis. A central site of inhibition of reponses to painful stimulation was seen in experimental studies in which locally administered dipyrone only slowly reduced firing of peripheral nerves in response to a knee inflammation, but given i.v. immediately blocked firing of neurones in the spinal cord. It is suggested that dipyrone acts in the spinal cord to exert its analgesic effect, possibly by inhibiting PG synthesis in nerve tissue.

Most NSAIDs are acidic and therefore accumulate within inflammatory lesions and are concentrated in the gastrointestinal tract, kidney and liver after oral administration. Inhibition of PG synthesis at these sites and in platelets contributes to the common adverse effects of NSAIDs, including gastrointestinal bleeding and renal dysfunction. Because of its non-acidic nature and weak inhibition of peripheral PG synthesis, dipyrone does not show the adverse events profile typical of NSAIDs.

In conclusion, dipyrone has a predominantly central analgesic action and a low gastrointestinal adverse event profile because of weak peripheral inhibition of PG synthesis.

Clinical pharmacokinetics of dipyrone and its metabolites

Professor M. Levy, M.D.
Jerusalem, Israel

Dipyrone is a water soluble compound which undergoes rapid hydrolysis in the gastrointestinal tract to the major active metabolite, 4-methyl-ami-no-antipyrine (MAA), following oral administration. Recent studies have shown that oral bioavailability of dipyrone tablets is 85%. Maximal plasma concentrations of MAA after oral dipyrone (0.75 g – 1.5 g) are achieved in 1–1.5 h and these kinetics are little affected by food.

In total, 20 different metabolites can be detected in humans, but 4 major metabolites account for two-thirds of the dipyrone dose. These are the 2 active metabolites, MAA and 4-amino-antipyrine (AA), together with the inactive metabolites 4-formyl-amino-antipyrine (FAA) and 4-acetyl-amino-antipyrine (AAA). The latter is formed by the hepatic N-acetyl-transferase system and is therefore subject to polymorphism, some subjects being slow and others fast acetylators. The mean elimination half-life of AA, consequently, varies from 3.8 h in fast to 5.5 h in slow acetylators (Fig. 1). Plasma kinetics of the metabolites are not completely linear, suggesting that over the 1 g – 3 g dose-range, saturation of metabolic enzymes may occur. Protein binding of all four metabolites is low.

"Dipyrone is a pro-drug which is hydrolysed to the active metabolites."

No ethnic differences in dipyrone pharmacokinetics are known. Clearance of dipyrone and its metabolites decreases slightly on multiple-dosing and with age and decreases significantly in liver cirrhosis. Renal impairment also reduces clearance but mainly of the inactive end metabolites. Interactions with cyclosporin A have been reported.

On the basis of the pharmacokinetic properties of dipyrone, it is considered that a four times daily regimen is justified. In view of its high therapeutic index, the recommended dose is 0.5 g to 1.0 g orally which takes into account the complex pharmacokinetics. Intravenous infusion administered slowly is preferred for rapid relief of colic pain at a recommended total dose of 1 g to 2 g dipyrone.

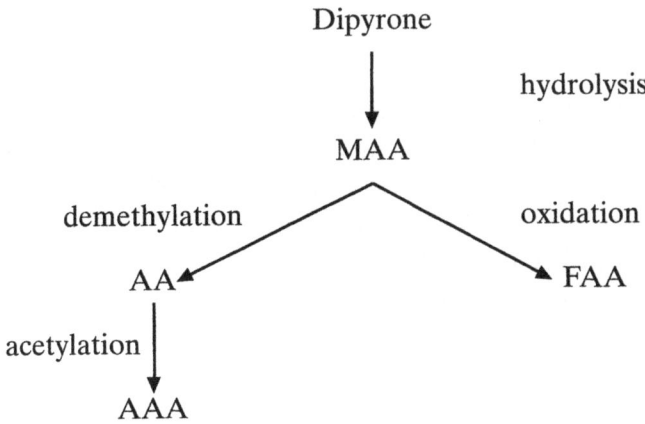

Fig. 1:
Metabolism of dipyrone
AA = 4-amino-antipyrine; AAA = 4-acetyl-amino-antipyrine; FAA = 4-formyl-amino-antipyrine; MAA = 4-methyl-amino-antipyrine

Dipyrone in acute postoperative and colic pain

C. Haag-Molkenteller, M.D.
Frankfurt/Main, Germany

Since its clinical introduction in 1922, dipyrone has become available in more than 100 countries throughout the world and has been the subject of more than 2000 publications. Here are the results of an evaluation of clinical acute pain studies published during the period 1973 to 1994, at a time when modern standards of clinical practice had already been introduced. The evaluation encompassed 33 studies in post-operative pain and 13 studies in renal colic and biliary pain. A total of 4766 patients were documented, including 2004 treated with dipyrone, the others with a reference drug or placebo.

"Dipyrone has a clear opioid-sparing effect ..... a fast onset of action and a broad therapeutic range, it has marked efficacy and there is no risk of addiction."

Effective drug treatment of acute pain requires a rapid onset and a duration of action longer than 1 h, the option of intravenous administration and the possibility of re-dosing. The meta-analysis of randomized, parallel group studies on single oral administration in 710 patients showed 0.5 g dipyrone to be an effective analgesic, with a faster onset of action at 1 g.

In post-operative pain of various etiologies, 1–2 g dipyrone administered by intravenous infusion provided rapid pain relief. Given orally, 0.5 g dipyrone provided greater pain relief than did 0.5 g paracetamol and was at least as effective as 0.5 g aspirin, which causes bleeding at higher doses. In renal colic, parenteral dipyrone provided a 60% reduction in pain against baseline within 15 min. The equal efficacy of doses of 1 g to 2.5 g dipyrone is attributed to the direct muscle relaxant action of the drug and suggests a ceiling in the dose-response effect. Importantly, both the muscle relaxant, N-butylscopolamine (hyoscine, 20 mg) and the opioid, tramadol (100 mg) were less effective than dipyrone. In several comparative studies in post-operative pain using patient-controlled analgesia (PCA), dipyrone was effective as the sole analgesic and provided the additional benefit of its opioid-sparing effect.

Adverse events associated with dipyrone administration were observed in 133 of 2004 patients; none were serious, consisting predominantly of nausea or vomiting. Interestingly, one suicide attempt was made with 100 g dipyrone without any adverse events. Adverse events associated with dipyrone given as PCA in patients with post-operative pain were significantly less than in patients receiving PCA-morphine or buprenorphine (Table 1).

Table 1:
Number of patients with adverse events during treatment of post-operative pain with dipyrone, morphine or buprenorphine given as patient-controlled analgesia.

Group[a]	Sedation	Vomiting	Pruritus	Pain on injection	Urine retention
	$(p=0.0001)$[b]	$(p=0.07)$[b]	$(p=0.02)$[b]	$(p=0.0002)$[b]	$(p=0.54)$[b]
Morphine	26 (52%)	13 (26%)	7 (14%)	0 (0%)	3 (6%)
Dipyrone	7 (14%)	6 (12%)	0 (0%)	8 (16%)	1 (2%)
Buprenorphine	24 (48%)	15 (30%)	3 (6%)	0 (0%)	3 (6%)

[a] n=50 per group. [b] dipyrone compared with morphine and buprenorphine
L.M. Torres et al. Rev. Esp. Anestesiol. Reanim. 1993; 40: 181–184.

It is concluded that dipyrone has at least comparable efficacy to tramadol, pethidine and non-steroidal anti-inflammatory drugs (NSAIDs) such as diclofenac in the treatment of acute pain. However, dipyrone treatment is not associated either with an increased risk of gastrointestinal or post-operative bleeding, as seen with NSAIDs, nor with an increased risk of psychological dysfunction, usually associated with opioids. Its additional spasmolytic properties make it particularly useful in colic pain.

Non-opioid analgesics in the treatment of acute pain

Professor S.A. Schug, M.D.
Auckland, New Zealand

Contrary to what might be expected, as many as 30–70% of post-operative patients have significant pain within the first 48 h after the operation. The reasons for this include the unpredictable variability of acute pain, based on incidence, intensity and time course, as well as the different patient characteristics. The modern armamentarium for the treatment of acute pain includes non-narcotic analgesics, opioids and local anesthetics. While opioids and local anaesthetics are the primary analgesic therapies for acute post-operative pain, the opioids have a very high side-effect profile, which is directly related to their mechanism of action. An average of 50–60% of patients suffer from nausea or vomiting with opioids. Respiratory depression can be reduced with patient-controlled analgesia, though it always remains a risk. Local anaesthetics must also be administered by skilled physicians, but are very useful for post-operative pain.

Among the non-opioid analgesics, paracetamol can provide suitable post-operative pain relief, particularly in day-stay surgery. It has few side-effects, nearly complete bioavailability and shows high patient acceptance, but is restricted by limited efficacy and the unavailability in most countries of a parenteral formulation. At doses above the therapeutic range it causes irreversible hepatotoxicity.

Non-steroidal anti-inflammatory drugs (NSAIDs) are useful in inflammatory pain and when soft tissues are involved, as in dental surgery. In day surgery, they have the advantage over opioids of not causing nausea or sedation. However, their use as opioid-sparing agents is of limited value unless the adverse effects associated with the administration of opioids are reduced as a result; this has not been shown conlusively as yet. The main limitation of NSAIDs is their potential to cause gastric injury, though on short-term administration such complications are unusual, as is perioperative bleeding due to inhibition of platelet aggregation. Nevertheless, because of the potential for bleeding, the use of NSAIDs in patients with hematological disorders is contraindicated. In patients with normal hydration, adverse effects of NSAIDs are not likely, but patients with hypotension, hydrovolemia, atherosclerosis, congestive heart failure, cirrhosis, renal insufficiency or diuretic treatment are predisposed to renal problems when taking NSAIDs. Ketorolac was withdrawn from some European markets for this reason.

"Dipyrone is more potent than paracetamol ..... and could play a role after minor and immediate surgery as the sole analgesic in day-stay surgery and in colic."

With an analgesic effect in post-operative pain comparable to that of opioids, its additional smooth muscle relaxing action and lack of NSAID-specific adverse effects, dipyrone is a very useful single analgesic in minor and intermediate surgery, day surgery, colic and in combination with regional analgesia. Its availability in a parenteral formulation is a big advantage over paracetamol, for instance. Additional clinical trial data are eagerly awaited. Several of the gaps in current post-operative pain management may be filled by dipyrone.

Comparative safety of analgesics

S.E. Andrade, Ph.D.
Rhode Island, USA

The non-opioid analgesics, dipyrone and paracetamol, have different safety profiles to those of the non-steroidal anti-inflammatory drugs (NSAIDs). The findings of an epidemiological analysis carried out on the safety of aspirin, diclofenac, paracetamol and dipyrone highlight these distinctions.

Studies published in English during the period 1970 to 1995 were reviewed. They included nine case-control studies, one each on agranulocytosis, aplastic anemia and anaphylaxis and seven studies on serious upper gastrointestinal bleeding (UGIB). These were restricted to reports of short-term (1 week) exposure to the analgesics. Safety was assessed by estimating the excess mortality calculated as the risk of mortality among patients with adverse events following subtraction of the risk in non-analgesic users.

"Excess mortality associated with dipyrone appears to be similar to paracetamol and is substantially lower than the risk of mortality due to gastrointestinal bleeding with NSAIDs."

As shown in table 1, the overall excess mortality estimate per 100 million users over a 1 week period was highest for the two NSAIDs, due to the much higher risk of death due to UGIB among these drugs. The slightly higher risk of agranulocytosis with dipyrone is minimal in relation to this risk of UGIB among NSAIDs, which was unaffected by the presence or absence of underlying gastrointestinal complications.

Drawing on the available data, it is concluded that dipyrone and paracetamol are both clearly associated with a much lower absolute risk of mortality due to adverse events than the NSAIDs for short-term therapy.

Table 1:
Excess mortality[a] estimates for short-term exposure to non-narcotic analgesics

	Aspirin	Diclofenac	Paracetamol	Dipyrone
Agranulocytosis	0.6	0	0.1	7.4
Aplastic amenia	0.3	5.4	0.6	0
Anaphylaxis	0.2	0.4	0.1	0.2
UGIB[b]	166	586	19	17
Overall excess mortality estimate per 100 million/week	167.2	591.5	19.8	24.7

[a] Expected number of deaths after subtracting the risk due to other possible causes than the drug itself.
[b] upper gastrointestinal bleeding.

In discussing these data, Dr. F. Michel (Frankfurt/Main) pointed out that, based on estimates in Germany, the costs of dipyrone, in terms of hospitalization due to adverse events, is 1–7 fold *less* than that of paracetamol and 7–10 fold less than that of diclofenac.

Routines, practice and needs for analgesics in out-patient surgery in Sweden

Professor N. Rawal, M.D., Ph.D.
Örebro, Sweden

Day-surgery on an ambulatory basis is widespread in the United States and becoming increasingly so within Europe. Main priorities in such patients are to maintain alertness, ambulation, analgesia and alimentation. In a recent national survey of over 1000 patients it was found that 64% of post-operative patients interviewed had mild pain, 25% moderate pain and 11% severe pain (mainly after inguinal hernia, skeletal surgery or breast surgery) on returning home. As many as 30% had difficulty in sleeping due to pain after surgery. This inadequate analgesia is sometimes responsible for unanticipated hospital re-admissions after surgery. In addition, nausea and vomiting delay discharge and are also responsible for unanticipated readmissions.

The nausea and vomiting is to some extent a result of the use of opioids for post-operative pain, which despite being the first choice for analgesia, have a high incidence of such adverse events. Alternatives are short-acting opioids (particularly in the recovery period) or regional analgesia which is associated with a low rate of complications. In 1995, 76% of Swedish anesthesiologists were using a spinal block for one-day surgery on inguinal hernia. Epidural analgesia is useful for surgery, because it keeps the patient alert and co-operative.

> "If this drug (dipyrone) is more potent than paracetamol with less side-effects than opioids we should use it frequently, it appears to be a pretty good drug."

It must be emphasized that pain management will only be as good as pain assessment, which should be carried out frequently using a visual analogue scale (hourly in ambulatory surgery or every 3h for in-patients) before and after surgery. This facilitates individual titration of analgesia, obviating the need for intramuscular treatment. Use of non-steroidal anti-inflammatory drugs (NSAIDs) for postoperative pain in day-stay surgery is on the increase. It is probably futile to attempt to reduce the requirement for opiates with NSAIDs, which may disparagingly be referred to as "New Sorts of Aspirin in Disguise". This is because, even at lower doses, opioids still exert adverse events which may be complicated by the gastric side-effects of NSAIDs. Paracetamol appears to be as effective as and safer than the NSAID ketorolac, for instance.

In the future, it is concluded that safe and simpler delivery systems will be required, with access to pre-packed analgesics, more ambulatory patient-controlled analgesia and better home-delivery analgesia. Dipyrone may provide a useful option between opioids and NSAIDs.

Perspectives

Even though it has a long history of use, dipyrone still offers distinct advantages over current analgesic therapies of acute pain. More potent than paracetamol, with a central site of action, dipyrone does not exhibit the adverse events typical of opioids (e.g. respiratory depression). It is also much less deleterious to the gastrointestinal mucosa than NSAIDs. Its unique direct spasmolytic activity is of additional advantage in colic pain.

With a rapid onset of action, and availability in an intravenous form, the drug can be re-dosed and offers a well-tolerated alternative to NSAIDs in the treatment of post-operative pain.

The re-introduction of dipyrone to Sweden exemplifies the confidence placed in the drug by physicians in many parts of the world.

GPSR Compliance

The European Union's (EU) General Product Safety Regulation (GPSR) is a set of rules that requires consumer products to be safe and our obligations to ensure this.

If you have any concerns about our products, you can contact us on ProductSafety@springernature.com

In case Publisher is established outside the EU, the EU authorized representative is:

Springer Nature Customer Service Center GmbH
Europaplatz 3
69115 Heidelberg, Germany

Batch number: 09636724

Printed by Printforce, the Netherlands